Biotin e-book

Contents

Introduction:

Vitamin B7, likewise called biotin, is a basic part of a healthy digestion system and making imperative chemicals within the human body. Biotin is frequently used to fortify hair and nails, and is likewise called vitamin H (for hair).

"Numerous frameworks in the human body take advantage from biotin including the skin, nerves, digestive tract, digestion system and cells," said Dr. Sherry Ross, obstetrician/ gynecologist and women's health expert at Providence Saint John's Health Center in Santa Monica, California. "Biotin is required for the development of unsaturated fats and glucose, which are utilized as vitality as a part of our body."

Biotin is found in little sums in food sources. "Foods that contain biotin are liver, cauliflower, salmon, carrots, bananas, soy flour, yeast, wheat germ, entire grain oats, entire wheat bread, eggs, dairy items, nuts, Swiss chard and chicken," said Ross.

Microscopic organisms in the small guts additionally make biotin, as per the University of Maryland Medical Center. This means that our body also produces biotin in small amounts. This shows that biotin is actually necessary for the well being of human body.

Medical advantages

Biotin is crucial to numerous body capacities. By University of Maryland Medical Center, vitamin B7 is utilized by the body to metabolize starches, fats and amino acids. It is likewise fundamental for the typical development of babies.

- Numerous individuals take biotin supplements to expand the strength of their skin, hair and nails. While more research is required, it appears that B7 might be useful in these zones. A twofold visually impaired study by the Ablon Skin Institute Research Center and the University of California found that taking biotin made huge hair development in ladies with transitory hair diminishing. The US National Library of Medicine additionally takes note of that biotin can be useful in the treatment of skin rashes in newborn children known as seborrheic dermatitis or support top. There is no exploration to demonstrate this case, as indicated by the Penn State Hershey Medical Center.

  "Biotin is essential for hair, skin and nails," said Lauren Graf, clinical dietitian for Montefiore-Einstein cardiac wellness program. "Low levels of biotin can give rise to fragile nails and diminishing hair. There is some proof that biotin supplements can reverse hair diminishing, particularly on the off chance that you are inadequate in taking the supplement. Taking a biotin supplement is not prone to be unsafe and might enhance hair quality."

- B7 might likewise be useful in the treatment of diabetes. A study by Alpha Therapy Center found that a treatment that joins chromium picolinate and B7 enhances glucose digestion system in patients with type 2 diabetes. High measurements of biotin were likewise discovered supportive in the treatment of fringe neuropathy, an indication of diabetes. Biotin assumes a noteworthy part in your blood glucose formation. Since biotin is intensely included in the breakdown of starches inside of your body, it is to a great extent in charge of keeping your glucose at healthy levels. On the off chance that you experience the ill effects of diabetes, you might be given a biotin supplement as an approach to get your glucose levels up to appropriately useful sums.

Dosage

Biotin inadequacy is uncommon in the United States. The few who don't get enough of this vitamin can have extremely detectable indications. "Insufficiency can bring about perplexity, sickness, muscle torment, skin changes and balding," Dr. Kristine Arthur, an internist at Orange Coast Memorial Medical Center in Fountain Valley, Canada, told Live Science. Different manifestations incorporate swollen and shaded tongue, dry eyes, splitting toward the sides of the mouth, weakness, loss of longing, sleep deprivation and despondency, as indicated by the University of Maryland Medical Center.

There are no official suggested day by day dosage rules for B7. Arthur recommends that grown-ups ought to go for 30 micrograms (mcg) every day. The Mayo Clinic prescribes 30 to 100 mcg for every day for grown-ups.

As a health knowledgeable individual, you as of now presumably realize that the b-complex vitamins assume a key part in metabolizing vitality, however you may not know as much about the activities of the individual b vitamins, for example, Biotin. You will likewise in some cases, hear biotin called either vitamin B7 or vitamin H. You have biotin present in your body actually, and it is extremely useful in a few of your real capacities, particularly those identified with your digestive system.

Biotin, alongside the other b-complex vitamins, has the primary elements of helping your body to process vitality, and of bringing carbon dioxide through your body. Your sweat organs, nerve tissue and bone marrow additionally work at their top proficiency when you have appropriate biotin levels.

You can likewise get other, much lesser known, profits by the biotin in your body or from the biotin that you ingest by means of supplements. Biotin supplements might be a possibility for you on the off chance that you might want to attempt to strengthen the constructive outcomes of this vitamin. While the primary reason that you would typically take a biotin supplement is to revise a biotin inadequacy, you can conceivably get other beneficial outcomes too.

Biotin is crucial for your metabolic procedure. This vitamin forms about each kind of foods that you ingest, including sugars, protein and fat. At the point when biotin levels are at the correct levels in your body, the food that you take in will be digested rapidly. Your specialist might even endorse a biotin supplement on the off chance that you experience the ill effects of metabolic issues, since it can get your digestive system up to ordinary working levels rapidly. In the event that you are attempting to get more fit, a biotin supplement might help, since it is infrequently thought to accelerate weight reduction, because of its reasonable impacts on metabolic levels.

Effects of biotin on skin:

Biotin is has very important effects on the skin, the vitamin is important for the proper breakdown and distribution of fatty acids which translates to healthy skin. Biotin deficiency has been shown to cause rash and dry itchy skin and generalized rash all over the body

Effects of biotin on liver:

Liver disease and a declining liver can be due to several causes, from infections like hepatitis to chronic liver failure and inherited causes, many liver diseases lead to deficiency of biotinidase leading to slow processing of biotin through the body and also decreased accumulation of biotin at cellular levels. Biotin deficiency also decreases glucokinase levels in liver resulting in decreased glycogen synthesis in liver. Biotin is also required for functioning of many liver enzymes that are responsible for generating energy molecules in our body.

Miscellaneous systemic effects of biotin:

Biotin also helps patients with high blood pressure, recent studies show that biotin can reduce thickening of arteries and reduce blood pressure in laboratory animals. Another study reveals that reduced intake of biotin in South African children lead to increased risk of hypertension in these children. Biotin along with chromium lowers the blood cholesterol levels and reduces the risk for hypertension and cardiovascular diseases.

It has also been shown that biotin maintains constant sugar levels in the blood, a function that is very important for people suffering from diabetes and also biotin intake also gives some relief to diabetic nerve pain as well.

Benefits of biotin on hair:

As mentioned before, it helps in the production of the human body's amino acids, as well as is a major drive in the formation of fatty acids. Keratin, a protein, also an essential component involved in the structure is made of amino acids. One should be aware that the building blocks of protein are basically constituted by amino acids.

Ever complained of rueful split ends and brittle hair or uneventful breakage of hair and premature graying of hair? Perhaps, it is what your hair need. Following are the benefits of biotin on all types of hair:

Biotin helps to promote hair growth since the structural components of this vitamin is similar to that of hair follicles. Also, it is recommended to take supplements orally since applying the substance directly onto the affected area may not be as effective as biotin's systemic formulae.

Biotin also helps to prevent breakage of hair as it strengthens the follicles, giving you a reason to flaunt the shine of your hair.

Biotin has been scientifically proven to help reverse the premature graying of hair.

One needs to ascertain to the biochemical aspects of the pigments of the hair which with age undergo specific modifications leading to the physiological graying of hair. Inadvertently, biotin is the supplement and the vitamin you need if you face premature graying of hair since it promotes the differentiation of the cells which are involved in the growth of follicles.

Biotin might have an essential part in the development and upkeep of your hair and nails. In the event that you experience the ill effects of a biotin lack, you will ordinarily encounter balding and fragile nails, and taking supplements of this vitamin might stop this procedure. By and large, taking a biotin supplement might even help you to grow new hair and nail development. Despite the fact that balding is once in a while created by a biotin inadequacy in your body, this issue can all the time be aided in the event that you take biotin supplements consistently. Regardless of the fact that you have ordinary biotin levels, you might take biotin as a supplement in the trusts of exploiting its capacity to animate fast hair and nail development.

Biotin general health benefits

Biotin, similar to the majority of the b-complex vitamins, has a vital part inside of your body. In the event that you think that you might be enduring a biotin lack, make a point to check with your specialist, and offer thought to a biotin supplement. Biotin offers your body considerably more than only a metabolic support - it can help practically all aspects of your body to accomplish and keep up great wellbeing.

There are no recorded symptoms for biotin in sums up to 10 milligrams a day, as per the Mayo Clinic. There is likewise no known dose of biotin that could bring about lethality in the body, bringing about overdose. Since all b vitamins are water dissolvable, the body does not store overabundance sums and flushes it away.

The word biotin originates from the old greek word "biotos," which signifies "life" or "sustenance." b vitamins, and particularly biotin, keep your skin, hair, eyes, liver, and sensory system solid. Biotin is additionally an essential supplement amid pregnancy, as it's vital for embryonic development.

A great many people get the biotin they require from eating a sound eating regimen, yet there have been numerous cases that getting more biotin can control your glucose, advance solid hair, skin and nails, and offer pregnant mothers some assistance with having more healthy children.

What amount of biotin is sufficient, where would you be able to get it, and what would it be able to truly accomplish for you?

Suggested daily amount

Somewhere around 30 and 100 mcg for each day of biotin are frequently prescribed for young people and grown-ups.

Since it's water-solvent, additional biotin will essentially go through your body when you urinate. While the vast majority can deal with biotin supplements, a few individuals report mellow reactions like queasiness and digestive issues. There are no known lethality indications connected with a lot of biotin.

Supplements and diabetes

Since a few studies demonstrate that individuals with type 2 diabetes have lower biotin levels, supplements might help with glucose regulation. The examination so far is clashed: a few studies demonstrate an impact when biotin is joined with chromium, while others don t.

Individuals with insulin-subordinate sort 1 diabetes likewise have a tendency to experience difficulty controlling their blood glucose levels. Biotin makes unsaturated fats by changing over glucose, and there is confirmation this can bring down glucose.

Healthy hair, skin, and nails

Biotin inadequacies are very common these days. But since individuals with an insufficiency frequently indicate manifestations of balding or a flaky red rash, a few specialists and supplement organizations prescribe expanding your intake of the supplement.

In any case, the National Institutes of Health (NIH) reports that there is inadequate information to bolster prescribing supplementation.

Fetal development

Biotin is likely protected on the off chance that you are pregnant or breastfeeding.

In any case, you ought to dependably let your specialist think about any supplements you are taking on the off chance that you are pregnant, breastfeeding, or might get to be pregnant.

Continuously check with your specialist before offering biotin to a child.

Biotin is additionally called vitamin H (the H speaks to Haar und Haut, German words for "hair and skin") or vitamin B7. Considers? on its bioavailability have been directed in rats and in chicks. In light of these studies, biotin bioavailability might be low or variable, contingent upon the kind of sustenance being devoured. All in all, biotin exists in nourishment as protein-bound structure or biocytin. Proteolysis by protease is required before assimilation. This procedure helps free biotin discharge from biocytin and protein-bound biotin. The biotin present in corn is promptly accessible; in any case, most grains have around a 20-40% bioavailability of biotin.

The wide variability in biotin bioavailability might be because of the capacity of a living being to break different biotin-protein bonds from sustenance. Whether a life form has a compound with that capacity will decide the bioavailability of biotin from the foodstuff.

A recent report distributed in the journal of nutrition reports that numerous pregnant ladies are biotin insufficient, and that pregnant mice with low biotin will probably have babies with serious birth imperfections. To advance infant wellbeing, specialists frequently suggest supplementing with biotin alongside folic acid amid pregnancy.

Characteristic sources of biotin

Biotin can likewise be found in various foods, including:

- Egg yolk
- Organ meats (liver, kidney)
- Nuts, similar to almonds, peanuts, pecans, and walnuts
- Nut spreads
- Soybeans and different vegetables

- Entire grains and oats
- Cauliflower
- Bananas
- Mushrooms

Since food preparing methods like cooking can render biotin ineffectual, raw or less-cooked variants of these foods contain more dynamic biotin.

The takeaway

While biotin is important for ordinary body capacity, and supplements might help pregnant women to have healthy babies without any sorts of deformities.

The human body contains an array of mineral compounds and vitamins that it needs so as to carry out normal functions of the body. Vitamins are required by our body in trace quantities. However, their role in maintaining cellular livability is too much crucial. It is only after years of discontinuing a particular vitamin intake that the body notices its absence and marks as deficient in lab reports.

A, b, c, d, e and k are the well-known vitamin compounds that are required by human body cells. Of these, vitamin a, d, e and k are fat-soluble, whereas the rest show solubility in liquid medium.

Let's glance at the roles of each of these vitamins in detail:

Vitamin A:

When it comes to immunity, maintenance of good vision, and proper growth and development of body structures, vitamin A plays a pivotal role. Retinol and beta-carotene are the two forms of this vitamin present widely in edible items.

Retinol when enters inside the body undergoes two important biological processes. It either converts into "retinoic acid", which is essential to keep up the health of skin, mineralization and re-mineralization processes of bones and teeth; growth of bone, etc. When retinol gets converted into "retinal", this compound becomes highly requisite for vision. Eggs and liver are rich sources of dietary retinol. Retinoid drugs are quite in use these days for the purpose of treatment of acne, scars and various other dermatological conditions.

[Warning: retinoic acid is not considered to be safe for use during pregnancy, as it harms the fetal growth and development].

Carotenoids are basically of the botanic origin and can be found in good quantities in carrots. The beautifully mesmerizing orange color of the autumn leaves is imparted by this compound. In the eye, carotene plays quite an important responsibility. Firstly, it acts as an antioxidant, and secondly, it absorbs the injurious UV and blue light from reaching the retina and the macula of the eyes (parts of the eyes with the most acute vision).

Deficiency of vitamin A in the body can lead to a famous pathology termed as 'night blindness'. Since aforementioned that both the forms of this compound are crucial for vision, hence it is quite apparent that their absence will leave the eye sight compromised.

Vitamin B complex:

The uses of vitamin b complex are mentioned under the heading "Biotin"

Vitamin C:

This compound is a famous anti-oxidant and is also known by the name of 'ascorbic acid'. It is made by many animals by their own body internally, with the exception of few species, namely the guinea pigs, most types of bats, as well as humans and monkeys. Without vitamin c, the body cannot carry out healing processes properly, which is well-explained in a condition termed as 'scurvy', in which, the gums bleed spontaneously and frequently owing to the absence of this organic compound in blood.

Ascorbic acids fights off oxidative stress quite efficiently, which is making it a popular agent in many anti-cancer drugs. Moreover, it plays a great role in the production of collagen and so, it being effectively incorporated into anti-aging medications. The repair process of wearing off tendons and ligaments, as well as iron absorption by blood cannot take place in the absence of this organic compound.

Green vegetables, citrus-containing foods, pineapples, papayas, watermelon, berry, red and green bell peppers; kiwi, tomatoes, potatoes and cantaloupes are some famous edible sources of vitamin c.

Vitamin D:

The term 'vitamin d' refers to a group of organic compounds that are fat-soluble sercosteroids (steroids with broken ring structure) chemically. Two essential forms of this vitamin exist in nature, namely cholecalciferol (d3) and ergocalciferol (d2) however the human body mostly makes use of the former type, which is also much more abundant as compared to the latter one. The absorption of calcium, magnesium, phosphate and zinc is carried out by vitamin d. Sunlight is the most rich and easily available source of the compound. However when it is absorbed by the skin, remain inactive until hydroxylated by enzymes present in the liver and kidneys. Hence, people with ailments concerning these two organs will also face deficiency of vitamin d if the illness is prolonged.

Since calcium absorption greatly depends upon the presence of this organic compound, vitamin D deficiency can lead to a condition termed as 'rickets', which is characterized by 'calcium-deficient weak bones and proximal muscle weakness' in children. A similar condition in adults is called as 'osteomalacia'.

Vitamin E:

These refer to a group of organic compounds namely tocopherols and tocotrienols. Just like vitamin c, vitamin e too is a powerful anti oxidant. Being fat soluble in nature, it gets incorporated into the fatty cell membrane layers, protecting them from radical specie damage. Alpha-tocopherol has the ability to suppress the enzymes that cause extra smooth muscle growth. By supporting the function of a growth factor ctgf (connective tissue growth factor), vitamin e helps in wound healing and repair. It also aids in maintaining cns functions and prevents platelet coagulation. Wheat oil, corn oil, sunflower oil, olive oil, avocados, papayas, pumpkin, broccoli, sesame oil asparagus and kiwi are some rich sources containing this anti-oxidant vitamin.

Vitamin K:

Here comes a really important vitamin which the nature has chosen to maintain blood dynamic. With the absence of vitamin k in the body, the process of coagulation and clot formation cannot initiate, as it is observed in people who are vitamin K deficient that their body becomes incapable of preventing blood leak from even wounds of even minor intensity. The compound can be divided into vitamin k1 and vitamin k2. Vitamin k 1 is basically found in plants, and hence is termed as phyllloquinone. Green leafy vegetables are stuffed with this compound. The second type of vitamin k is known as menaquinone.

Kiwi, cabbages, lettuce, turnips, broccoli, mustard, kale, swiss chard, collards, brussels, cauliflower, grapes, and avocado are some famous sources of vitamin k that are available easily.

Uses of vitamin b in the human body

Before we head on towards the health benefits of biotin, let us discuss in detail the role and contributions of vitamin b complex in the human body.

There are a total of 8 kinds of vitamin b in nature, which are described in detail as under:

Vitamin B1:

It is also known as 'thiamine'. It is naturally synthesized in bacteria, fungi and plants, but not in humans, who must obtain it in their diet, and hence this vitamin is termed as an essential nutrient. The most concentrated food sources of thiamin are pork and yeast extracts. Rye, sunflower seeds, oat, cauliflower, kale, liver, potatoes and oranges are some other useful sources as well. Thiamine deficiency casts some potentially fatal effects in the body such as the "beri beri", which is a disease of the cardiovascular and neurological systems. Wernicke-korsakoff syndrome is another serious medical condition that arises owing to vitamin b1 deficiency.

Vitamin B2:

It is also known as ribloflavin. Cofactors in the body, that is, fad and fmn, two vital members of the electron transport chain family, that work to carry out the most important functions at cellular level, including respiration, make use of this vitamin. Riboflavin can be obtained from foods such as cheese, kidneys, legumes, yeast, milk, mushrooms, almonds, and liver. Ariboflavinosis is a condition referred to deficiency of riboflavin in blood. Stomatitis and angular stomatitis are some important signs of the disease. Moreover, a lack of vitamin b2 in the body can cause scaly rashes on the body, and may also produce anemia.

Vitamin B3:

It is also known as niacin. Currently, this type of organic compound is being employed by pharmaceutical companies as well as supplemental brands for the purpose of treatment of hypercholesterolemia. Niacin deficiency in body is termed as 'pellagra', and it produces certain symptoms such as anemia, mouth lesions, nausea, headache, skin lesions and tiredness. Vitamin b 3 can be found in several foods such as asparagus, carrots, sweet potatoes, fish, chicken, liver, beef, kidney, heart, legumes, nuts, whole grains, broccoli, leafy vegetables, mushrooms, dates, and avocados.

Vitamin B5:

It is also known as pantothenic acid. Vitamin b 5 is also an essential nutrient, that is, it cannot be synthesized by the human body, and must be obtained from diet. Some skin and hair products make use of this vitamin as an ingredient. Coenzyme a (coa) is a compound that is used by the body cells so as to synthesize fatty acids and cholesterol. Patothenic acid is used to synthesize this coa. Meat is the biggest source of this vitamin. Whole grains, avocado, broccoli, rice, mushroom, and wheat bran are some other rich sources of pantothenic acid. Its deficiency is extremely rare, but when occurs, produces symptoms similar to those observed in ariboflavinosis.

Vitamin B6:

It is also known as pyridoxine. Bananas, chickpeas, turkey, potatoes, pistachios, beef and pork are some good food sources of vitamin b6. Its deficiency can lead to angular glossitis, seborrhoeic dermatitis, conjunctivitis, intertrigo, confusion, and neuropathy.

Vitamin B7:

It is also known as biotin, vitamin h or coenzyme r. This vitamin acts as a cofactor that aids in carbon dioxide transfer at several enzymatic functions in the body. Amino acid catabolism, gluconeogenesis and fatty acid synthesis are some vital functions that require the presence of biotin. Liver, raw egg yolk, egg whites, peanuts, green leafy veggies, and Swiss chard are few useful sources of biotin. Hair loss, lethargy, numbness, conjunctivitis and dermatitis are few symptoms that occur due to the deficiency of vitamin b7..

Vitamin B9:

It is also known as folic acid or vitamin m. Folic acid is very important for human blood, and frequent supplement intake of folic acid is a high requirement during pregnancy. Its deficiency usually occurs during gestation, and may lead to symptoms such as forgetfulness, depression, weakness, lethargy, swelling of tongue, headache, irritability, palpitations, confusion and shortness of breath. Brussels, avocado, green leafy vegetables, yeast, liver, spinach, seafood, meat, and eggs are few useful sources of vitamin b9.

Vitamin B12:

It is also known as cyanocobalamin or hydroxocobalamin. It is a vitamin component of the CNS system, and is important for the maintenance of neurological functions of the body. Poor memory, depression, confusion and fatigue are some common symptoms produces due to its deficiency. In extreme cases, symptoms of more serious intensity such as mania and psychosis can also occur. Vitamin b12 deficiency also leads to a condition known as 'megaloblastic anemia', in which the rbcs are bigger than usual. Meat, fish, poultry, egg whites and egg yolks are some common sources of this compound.

How does biotin boost your health?

Ever wondered why biotin is also called as vitamin H? To what has been mentioned above, one needs to understand the entire concept behind the uses and the benefits of Ourand? why it has been named pivotally as vitamin H. Germans are not only known notoriously for Hitler or the Nazis, but gladly, two terms of its language made it to medicine as well. 'Haar', translated as 'hair', and haut translated as 'skin' have been the terms responsible for the h lagging behind this vitamin's name.

This eBook caters to private label biotin's most essential features, those of which revolve mainly around its benefits and issues related to its deficits, loss of supplementation and healthcare production.

Vitamins are very important nutrients that are required by all of us in minute quantities to function properly, more importantly vitamins are responsible for a lot of reactions that are going inside our body, from the construction of new cells, to tissue growth and antioxidant effects, they are vital for enzymes to function in our body. They have diverse biochemical function from making bones stronger to increasing immunity against certain diseases. Vitamins are part of our daily diet, most of us take vitamins from food and dietary sources, and during deficiency we might take vitamins in the form of supplements, supplements are very important form of vitamin intake. At present 13 vitamins are known. Vitamins are classified according to their physiological and biochemical activity and not their chemical structure. Vitamins are extremely important for normal growth and development throughout the person's life.

Vitamin B complex (from B1-B12) are water soluble vitamins, is an important vitamin complex, that play central role in important body's function, the vitamins help in metabolism of fat, carbohydrate and protein and also help in generating energy for the body's function. Deficiencies of these vitamins lead to array of pathologies from dermatitis, hair fall, and diarrhea, anemia to psychosis, mania, dementia and death, thus highlighting the importance of vitamin intake in our daily life.

Of this complex vitamin B7, also known as biotin or simply vitamin h is of utmost importance, not a true vitamin, since it's manufactured by intestinal flora, it is water soluble. Biotin is utilized by various systems of the body like skin, nails, nervous system and digestive tract. ~~Biotin~~ It is also needed for metabolism of fatty acids and glucose. Biotin is a crucial vitamin during pregnancy and essential for fetal growth.

The recommended daily intake of biotin is 30mcg/day. However the daily requirement for pregnant woman is 35mcg/day. Biotin deficiency is common. The daily requirement of biotin is quite small, and usually fulfilled by our daily diet, and intestinal bacteria synthesizes small amounts of it, however deficiencies can be caused by consuming raw egg whites over a period of months to years. Eggs contain avidin that binds to biotin and when eggs are excessively cooked avidin is lost. Biotin deficiency can occur in number of other cases as well, like a person who's on total parenteral diet, ketogenic diet and protein deficiency as well. Drugs have important role to play, and sometime effect biotin metabolism and absorption. Severe malnutrition, smoking, alcohol consumption and excessive anti-diuretic intake also play a role in biotin deficiency. Low levels of biotin in infants leads to hair loss and seborrheic dermatitis. Symptoms of deficiency of biotin are greatly improved by intake of biotin via supplements.

Irrespective of the aforementioned features, biotin also helps in the maintenance of a healthy relationship with your hair. Nowadays, there are a lot of shampoos which owe their success mainly due to the administration of biotin as vitamin h in their ingredients. Not only shampoos, many other hair products such as conditioners and hair setting sprays have also been proven to benefit from biotin in their complex commercially.

Let's discuss the needs of the scalp in relation to some of the world's easily attainable protein foods. Not only proteins, but you need to know how to take care of your scalp as well. Apples, carrots, eggs and milk are the major foods that every scalp needs to be taken care of. These foods are easily available during all seasons and in every continent of the world as well.

Following are some life hacks which your scalp may benefit from in addition to biotin:

- Keep in mind that your scalp needs nutrients for the hair to flourish. Some of the major nutrients are present in your everyday foods, which include dairy products, fruits, nuts such as almonds and green beverages which contain high amounts of biotin.

- Body stress has to be adequately maintained. Mental stress levels and body perspiration can be controlled if one caters to green beverages such as green tea after an eventful exercise leading to perspiration and sweat. These specific drinks are high in vitamins including vitamin B complex and may lead to an appropriately functioning system.

Consider feeding your hair with biotin in the form of Oursupplements? for better growth and maintenance of texture of your hair. One should also keep in mind that latest researches are supportive of the fact that biotin's deficiency may lead to brittle or breakage of hair.

Benefits of biotin on nails:

One would deem Ourto? be a lifesaver as it has benefits not only for your hair, but also for your skin, nails and a couple of your internal organs. Did you know that vitamins help in the maintenance of metabolism of the body? Biotin is one of those vitamins, which caters to the chaos evident in the brittleness of the nails. Biotin also prevents the chipping of the nails, and may also serve to strengthen the cuticles hand in hand.

Supplementation:

Ideally, biotin is accompanied by other vitamins and minerals when prepared in the form of oral supplementations. However, one must keep in mind that different multivitamins containing biotin as its essential component may differ in its dosage and efficacy.

Biotin supplements are also used in number of congenital metabolic disorders such as biotinidase deficiency, multiple carboxylase deficiency, and holocarboxylase synthetase deficiency can also lead to inborn or late-onset forms of biotin deficiency. In all these forms of metabolic enzyme deficiencies biotin supplements play an important role in keeping individuals body functioning normal.

For instance, there are a lot of medicines which contain vitamin b supplements in its complex such as vitamin B7, riboflavin, vitamin B12 and others. Some may also contain calcium and iron within their oral capsules. Oral supplements are always preferred as many other compounded foods may also contain artificial components which may not be equivalent to deficit of the vitamin in the body.

One should also keep this in mind that different forms of supplementations vary in their dosages. One form of supplements may not be as effective as another form of supplements just because of mere differences in their amounts quantity and presence of artificial toxins.

Let's consider a salient feature which forms the backbone of these supplements – all of these supplements provide the person with adequate synergy, including positive effects in metabolism relating to the brain, nerves and adequate bodily monitoring.

Biotin supplementations are also used along with some drugs, since sometimes drugs alter the metabolism of biotin. Anti-convulsants like phenytoin carbamazipine cause biotin deficiency and increase its catabolism, these drugs cause reduced intestinal absorption and renal absorption of biotin, leading to reduced biotin concentration in the blood. Therefore for someone on long term anti convulsant therapy, increased intake of biotin is very important. People on long term antibiotic therapy alter the intestinal flora and hence need enhanced intake of biotin.

Biotin is essentially a very important vitamin and its deficiency causes several problems, regular intake of biotin through diet or alternatively through supplements must be ensured

Effects of biotin in chronic smokers

Minimal research is suggestive of the cons of smoking on biotin, however, studies are suggestive of the fact that chronic smokers may suffer from an obscure deficiency of biotin, especially if they are suffering from chronic obstructive pulmonary disease.

Smoking is another main health problem faced by national healthcare of many countries, while smoking itself is harmful; it also leads to multi vitamins deficiency, like biotin. Smokers catabolize biotin much more rapidly than non smokers; a study provides evidence of accelerated biotin metabolism in smoker women, which results in marginal biotin deficiency. Biotin helps smokers by getting rid of toxin build up in the body; it also increases the production of hair cells. Biotin also helps keep the capillaries of skin open and provides some essential nutrients to your hair, skin, and nails.

Effects of biotin on pregnant women:

Pregnancy is a physiological condition in which nutritional demand of several vitamins increase, one such vitamin is biotin, deficiency of biotin in mother and fetus during pregnancy has been of great interest in researchers, since in mammals, the deficiency of vitamin is a tetragonic event. Approximately 50% women show increased excretion of 3-hia, indicating deficiency of vitamin H/biotin. Hence biotin supplements are sometimes given to pregnant women with established biotin deficiencies.

Many studies, back in 2009, were supportive of the fact that many pregnant women face consult their doctors mainly due to striking symptoms such as facial rash which were suggestive of a deficiency in vitamin B H, also known as biotin. Many pregnant women complain of symptoms related to deficiencies of folic acid, iron or biotin.

During pregnancy, metabolism of our major vitamins and minerals become two or three fold due to its requirements in the body. Nevertheless, one should keep this in mind that illnesses during the third trimester of pregnancy can be prevented if a pregnant woman caters to Ourfrom? the start of her pregnancy. The dosages may vary. However, pregnant women are usually recommended 30 mcg of biotin as a daily ritual, which would help prevent congenital defects as well such as cleft palate and lip.

Effects of biotin in chronic alcoholics:

Alcohol inhibits the transport of vitamin B12 as well as biotin across the intestinal junction. Most of the digestion and absorption in the human body takes place from the small intestines. Alcohol reportedly inhibits the cofactors necessary for the transport of biotin across the walls of the intestine, providing a supportive reason relating to the deficiency of biotin in chronic alcoholics. Physiologic concentration of biotin may lack in the body of an alcoholic, even if the oral intake is up to mark and supposedly fulfilling.

Alcoholism is an addiction that many suffer from, alcoholism not only causes social imparity but it has profound physical effects as well, one such effect is decreased absorption of biotin in small intestine and decreased uptake in the large intestine and storage in the body. Chronic alcohol use in humans is associated with a significant reduction in plasma biotin levels, and animal studies have shown inhibition in intestinal biotin absorption by chronic alcohol feeding. At cellular levels chronic alcohol consumption leads to slower entry of biotin in the cells of the body. Alcoholics may present with number of signs and symptoms of biotin deficiency for example skin rash to psychosis to parenthesis and infection. One of the major parts of physical recovery of alcoholics is taking supplements to eliminate deficiency of important nutrient and biotin supplement is an important part of nutrition in addiction recovery.

Effects of biotin on weight:

As excitement surpasses the line, we now know that biotin has a lot of positive effects on the body. Whereas it may benefit the skin in getting rid of acne, it also has benefits in the maintenance of weight and the body mass. In order to keep your body mass index along the line, you need to cater to biotin and see its magic as its helps you to get rid of the excessive carbohydrates that have been piled up in storage in excess in your body.

Correct supplements of Biotin, as we manufacture, may help you tone your body by metabolizing the carbohydrates into energy which can be used for important functions in the body.

Personal experiences:

Our biotin has been in the market for a long period of time. We not only provide you with supplements related to vitamin b complex, but provide you a wide range of medicines to choose from, depending on your need, time and prescription, of course.

In this case, Biotin manufactured by us had considered catering to a couple of individuals who were facing troubles with brittle nails, obscure texture and too much breakage of hair and rash on facial skin. Our Biotin has been fortunate enough to meet with its customers requirements. Many doctors place patients who complain of sudden break outs of acne on two years or more for optimum results. Many individuals have also complained of the drying effects of shampoos which lead to brittle hair. With our in the market, and also in the human system, these individuals have stopped complaining since they have regained confidence as their hair and skin continue to shine even without the use of any beauty regimens which usually recommend otherwise.

Since biotin is a solute which is easily soluble in water, it is recommended to drink lots of water with it for optimum efficacy. Nevertheless, biotin does not get piled up in the body or goes into waste due to its solubility. Prescriptions usually start from little amounts of dosages which may work up their way to large amounts after a period of time.

Biotin Side Effects

Biotin is a sheltered and nontoxic vitamin. It has not been connected with any genuine symptoms, even in extensive dosages.

The FDA reports that biotin is safe and very much endured when taken by mouth in suggested dosages.

Elements that influence biotin requirements

The recurrence of negligible biotin status is not known, but rather the occurrence of low flowing biotin levels in people has been observed to be much more prominent than in the all inclusive community. Additionally, moderately low levels of biotin have been accounted for in the pee or plasma of patients who have had a fractional gastrectomy or have different reasons for achlorhydria, blaze patients, epileptics, elderly people, and athletes. Pregnancy and lactation might be connected with an expanded interest for biotin. In pregnancy, this might be because of a conceivable speeding up of biotin catabolism, though, in lactation, the higher interest has yet to be clarified. Late studies have indicated minimal biotin lack can be available in human incubation, as confirmed by expanded urinary discharge of 3-hydroxyisovaleric corrosive, diminished urinary discharge of biotin and bisnorbiotin, and diminished plasma centralization of biotin. Furthermore, smoking might assist quicken biotin catabolism in women.

Deficiency

Biotin lack can emerge because of different characteristic hereditary blunders that influence the action of biotin-related chemicals. Subsequent to endogenous biotin creation happens in the gut, dysbiosis could likewise irritate the metabolic procedures that permit the body to produce biotin all alone.

The primary showing of biotin lack in humans was seen in creatures used raw egg white?. Rats encouraged egg white proteins were found to create dermatitis, alopecia and neuromuscular brokenness. This disorder, called egg white harm, was found to be brought on by a glycoprotein found in egg white, avidin. Avidin denatures after warming. This protein ties to a great degree well with biotin, making it distracted for use in enzymatic reactions.

Insufficiency side effects include:

- Male pattern baldness (alopecia)

- Conjunctivitis

- Dermatitis as a layered, red rash around the eyes, nose, mouth, and genital zone.

- Neurological indications in grown-ups, for example, anxiety, dormancy, and shivering of the extremities

The neurological and mental indications can happen with just small deficiencies. Dermatitis, conjunctivitis, and balding will for the most part happen just when lack deficiency out to be more serious. In serious instances of inadequacy, a trademark facial rash, together with an irregular facial fat dispersion, might likewise be seen (this has been termed the "biotin-insufficient face" by a few specialists) (no reference given).

People with genetic issue of biotin inadequacy have proof of impeded resistant framework capacity, including expanded weakness to bacterial and parasitic infections.

Pregnant ladies have a tendency to have a high danger of biotin inadequacy. About portion of pregnant ladies have strange expansions of 3-hydroxyisovaleric corrosive, which reflects diminished status of biotin. Several studies have reported this conceivable biotin lack amid the pregnancy might bring about newborn children's intrinsic distortions, for example, congenital fissure. Mice nourished with dried raw egg to affect biotin lack amid the pregnancy brought about up to 100% occurrence of the newborn children's malnourishment. Newborn children and incipient organisms are touchier to the biotin lack. Subsequently, even a mellow level of the mother's biotin insufficiency that does not achieve the presence of physiological inadequacy signs might bring about a genuine outcome in the newborn children.

Metabolic disorders

Acquired metabolic issue described by inadequate exercises of biotin-ward carboxylases is termed various carboxylase lack. These incorporate insufficiencies in the proteins holocarboxylase synthetase or biotinidase. Holocarboxylase synthetase insufficiency keeps the body's cells from utilizing biotin viably, and in this manner meddles with various carboxylase reactions. Biochemical and clinical signs include: ketolactic acidosis, natural aciduria, hyperammonemia, skin rash, sustaining issues, hypotonia, seizures, formative postponement, alopecia, and unconsciousness.

Biotinidase deficiency is not because of insufficient biotin, but instead to an inadequacy in the chemicals that produce it. Biotinidase catalyzes the cleavage of biotin from biocytin and biotinyl-peptides (the proteolytic debasement results of each holocarboxylase) and in this manner reuses biotin. It is additionally critical in liberating biotin from dietary protein-bound biotin. General manifestations incorporate diminished voracity and development. Dermatologic indications incorporate dermatitis, alopecia, and achromotrichia (nonattendance or loss of shade in the hair). Perosis (a shortening and thickening of bones) is found in the skeleton. Greasy liver and kidney disorder and hepatic steatosis additionally can occur.

Use in biotechnology

Biotin is broadly utilized all through the biotechnology business to conjugate proteins for biochemical assays. Biotin's little size means the organic movement of the protein will in all probability be unaffected. This procedure is called biotinylation. Since both streptavidin and avidin tie biotin with high fondness (Kd of $10-14$ mol/l to $10-15$ mol/l) and specificity, biotinylated proteins of diversion can be detached from a specimen by misusing this very steady association. The example is brooded with streptavidin/avidin dots, permitting catch of the biotinylated protein of diversion. Whatever other proteins tying to the biotinylated atom will likewise stay with the dot and all other unbound proteins can be washed away. Notwithstanding, because of the ? to a great degree, solid streptavidin-biotin collaboration, extremely brutal conditions are expected to elude the biotinylated protein from the dabs (ordinarily 6M guanidine HCl at pH 1.5), which frequently will denature the protein of diversion. To go around this issue, globules conjugated to monomeric avidin can be utilized, which has a diminished biotin-tying fondness of ~$10-8$ mol/l, permitting the biotinylated protein of enthusiasm to be eluted with abundance free biotin.

ELISAs regularly make utilization of biotinylated optional antibodies against the antigen of interest, trailed by a discovery step utilizing streptavidin conjugated to a journalist atom, for example, horseradish peroxidase or basic phosphatase.

Toxicity

Human researches have demonstrated few, if any, impacts because of abnormal state measurements of biotin. This might give proof of the fact that both individuals and people could endure dosages of no less than a request of size more prominent than each of their nutritious necessities. There are no reported instances of antagonistic impacts from accepting high measurements of the vitamin, specifically, when utilized as a part of the treatment of metabolic issue creating sebhorrheic dermatitis in infants. Excess biotin gathering can restrain endogenous sirt action prompting expanded irritation, cellularity, and collagen testimony and might be mostly in charge of age related metabolic issues.

Likely Effective for:

Treating and counteracting biotin deficiency. Side effects of deficiency incorporate diminishing of the hair (regularly with loss of hair shading), and red layered rash around the eyes, nose, and mouth. Different side effects incorporate discouragement, laziness, mental trips, and shivering in the arms and legs. There is some confirmation that cigarette smoking might bring about mild biotin lack.

Potentially Ineffective for:

- Skin rash in newborn children (seborrheic dermatitis).

Inadequate Evidence for:

Male pattern baldness. There is some preparatory proof that balding can be decreased when biotin is taken by mouth in blend with zinc while a cream containing the concoction compound clobetasol propionate (Olux, Temovate) is connected to the skin.

Diabetes. Biotin alone doesn't appear to influence glucose levels in individuals with type 2 diabetes. Be that as it may, there is some proof that a mix of biotin and chromium (Diachrome, Nutrition 21) may bring down glucose in individuals with diabetes, whose diabetes is inadequately controlled by professionally prescribed pharmaceuticals. Other early confirmation demonstrates that the same mix lessens proportions of aggregate cholesterol levels to "great" high-thickness lipoprotein (HDL) cholesterol, "awful" low-thickness lipoprotein (LDL) cholesterol to HDL cholesterol, and non-HDL to HDL cholesterol in individuals with type 2 diabetes.

Diabetic nerve torment. There is some confirmation that biotin can lessen nerve torment in individuals with diabetes.

Weak fingernails and toenails. Biotin may build the thickness of fingernails and toenails in individuals with fragile nails.

Different conditions. Today, vitamins and supplements are a multi-billion dollar industry, yet few individuals have even known about Vitamin H. Long known for its advantages to hair and skin, it is nothing unexpected that it has been alluded to as the "excellence vitamin." Otherwise known as Biotin, Vitamin B7 or Ccenzyme R, Vitamin H is a water-dissolvable B-complex vitamin whose advantages go more than shallow. Since it is moderately uncommon to be inadequate in this vitamin, researchers found the significance of Biotin rather unintentionally.

Investigations on humans which were nourished just raw egg whites created skin rashes and balding. When they added the yolks back to their eating routine, the side effects left. Obviously, something in the raw egg whites was bringing on the skin to get dry and disturbed and the hair to thin and shed. The same remained constant for individuals who devoured raw egg whites for a drawn out stretch of time or were tube-sustained through IV infusions without Biotin supplementation. Scientists found that there is a specific protein in raw egg whites called Avidin, which ties to Biotin, making it distant for ingestion by the body. Once the egg whites are cooked, the proteins break down, or "denature," and this is no more an issue for Biotin preparing. So obviously, Biotin is vital for legitimate working of skin and hair. In any case, many years of examination on Biotin has uncovered that it is likewise essential for the correct working of the sensory system and musculature and in keeping up cell forms like development, digestion system and vitality.

How Does Biotin Work?

Biotin is a critical segment of the catalysts that separates fats, sugars and different substances, changing over food into energy. Through these activities, Biotin can keep up relentless glucose levels and backing the sensory system. Biotin's impact on fat digestion system might truth is told by the way to comprehend the skin and hair issues found in Biotin deficiency. Since Biotin is required for the working of catalysts intended to deliver fat in the body, an inadequacy in Biotin will without a doubt influence fat preparing. This might seem like something to be thankful for, however it is entirely adverse with regards to the sensitive equalization of unsaturated fats in cells, for example, the skin cells that kick the bucket and are supplanted rapidly. Being the biggest organ in contact with nature, the skin likewise depends on unsaturated fats to shape a defensive boundary. Thus, skin cells give off an impression of being the first to hint at Biotin lack, bringing about dry skin and a disabled boundary against nature.

Signs of deficiency:

- Red, layered rash around the nose, mouth and eyes.
- Diminishing hair, at times with shedding and loss of shade (turning gray hair).
- Conceivable anxiety, weakness, depression.
- Shivering sensations in the arms and legs.
- Muscle spasms after activity.
- Conceivable elevated cholesterol and heart issues.
- Support top, a sort of seborrheic dermatitis of the scalp, head and eyebrows. In infants, dried up yellowish-whitish patches show up in these zones and could possibly be irritated.
- Expanded danger for creating other wellbeing issues

Where Can We Find It?

Like all B-vitamins, Biotin (B7) is water-solvent and is not put away in greasy tissues. So given its significance in keeping up a solid body, we should supplement with outer wellsprings of Biotin. B7 can be made by microscopic organisms, yeasts, molds, green growth and a few plants. Fortunately, we have a lot of intestinal microscopic organisms in our bodies that produce the important levels of this vitamin. A few studies demonstrate that upwards of 50 percent of pregnant ladies might be inadequate in Biotin, so supplementation amid pregnancy and smart nourishing can ~~demonstrate~~ be valuable for mother and child. Long haul utilization of anti-toxins or awkwardness in intestinal issues might annihilate these useful microorganisms, and we should look to nourishment hotspots for B7. Dietary hotspots for Biotin are various and ample, found in peanuts, liver, egg yolks, bananas, mushrooms, cauliflower, watermelon, vegetables and above all else Swiss chard. Brewer's yeast is another rich wellspring of Biotin. It is uplifting news for the individuals who appreciate an icy brew or Vegemite on toast (for our Australian neighbors). Since it is effectively accessible in like manner nourishment sources, there is no suggested dietary stipend (RDA) built up for Biotin in the U.S., and Biotin lack has a tendency to be mellow and bizarre. In any case, handled nourishments might demolish Biotin and different supplements, so unless you eat an assortment of entire foods, you may not be completely getting Biotin's medical advantages. Pregnant ladies might require more, however in the event that you are considering taking Biotin supplementation, converse with a doctor before rolling out any dietary improvements. Vitamin H, Biotin, B7 – whatever you call it – is actually an important part of keeping up a working body. So eat your entire products of the soil to profit by this vitamin you presumably did not know you require.

Vitamin H helps the body to process vitality and delivers carbon dioxide in the body. Keeping up appropriate level of vitamin H will help in legitimate working of sweat organs, bone marrow, and nerve tissue.

Vitamin H is additionally crucial for sound hair, liver, eyes, and skin solid. Absence of this vitamin can prompt wretchedness, dermatitis, male pattern baldness, sickliness, heart issues, elevated cholesterol and queasiness.

What is Biotin and Will it Make My Hair Grow Longer?

Intrigued by utilizing biotin supplements for more, more grounded hair? Begin with 1,250 mcg at mealtime, twice every day.

Before I dive into the low down insights about biotin supplements, let me clear about this first: I am not a specialist nor a doctor, so all that I am discussing here and the exhortation I give is just in light of my own encounters, assessments, and exploration, so before you choose to take a day by day dosage of biotin, make a point to counsel with your doctor.

Presently, What Is Biotin?

As mentioned many times in the book, Biotin is otherwise called vitamin H or B7. It is a water-solvent B-complex vitamin. Biotin supplements are regularly suggested for individuals with lacks of this vitamin to balance male pattern baldness.

Numerous individuals likewise take the supplement to build their hair development rate, and the outcomes differ from one individual to the next relying upon a few metabolic elements.

There are distinctive sentiments out there, however this is the thing that I have found: A substantial number of individuals report that biotin offers their common hair some assistance with growing speedier and more grounded (thicker). Despite the fact that biotin is accessible through specific nourishments (cooked eggs, sardines, nuts, entire grains, cauliflower, and mushrooms to give some examples), it is additionally actually created by our bodies. By expanding the dosage, we invigorate our bodies to make and develop hair and skin cells, making our hair more advantageous and more inexhaustible.

Presently, I ought to say right here that there are relatively few great studies demonstrating that biotin works. Here is one study by the University of Maryland Medical Center that essentially says the confirmation that biotin enhances fragile hair is powerless.

All things considered, the concentrate additionally says that biotin has not been connected with reactions, even in high measurements, and is thought to be non-poisonous.

So I take that to imply that we can attempt it and discover for ourselves on the off chance that it works for us.

What day by day dosage of biotin will offer your hair some assistance with growing longer and more grounded? The short reply: Start with 2,500 mcg day by day.

Take half (1,250 mcg) with breakfast and another 1,250 with supper for two weeks.

Audits of Biotin for Hair Growth

Biotin supplements can be a piece of a solid hair regimen, alongside a decent eating routine and a lot of water.

Biotin supplements can be a piece of a sound hair regimen, alongside a decent eating routine and a lot of water.

In the wake of experiencing a few hair development gatherings, here is the thing that I have observed: There is by all accounts a general accord that beginning with a low measurement of 2,500 mcg day by day helps a greater part of ladies expand their hair's development. Take half (1,250 mcg) with breakfast and the other half with supper for two weeks. Beginning with this these measurements and drinking bunches of water will offer your body some assistance with adjusting to the supplement.

Following two weeks, step by step expand the measurements until you are taking 5,000 mcg day by day (2,500 mcg with breakfast; 2,500 mcg with supper).

A few individuals report taking 10,000 mcg dosages day by day with great results, while others see comparative results with half of those measurements. You ought to see with your own eyes by expanding your dose steadily, making a point to record the advancement of your hair development taking pictures and estimations.

Following two weeks taking 2,500 mcg, bit by bit expand the measurement to 5,000 mcg absolute: 2,500 mcg with breakfast and 2,500 mcg with supper.

Results and Benefits of Using Biotin

Begin with 1,250 mcg of biotin supplement at mealtimes and work up to 2,500 mcg twice day by day for more, more grounded hair.

The rate that your hair will develop after you begin taking biotin supplements relies on upon a few elements: your digestion system (how rapidly you process and process supplements and sustenance), your day by day action level, your eating regimen, and how much water you drink.

In the event that you choose to attempt biotin to make your hair longer and more grounded, don't begin with a high measurement (a few locales prescribe taking 10,000 mcg to begin) and recollect: mcg implies microgram. That one millionth of a gram! A full gram of biotin would be 1,000,000 mcg!

When you start taking biotin supplements, you will probably see these advantages:

- more beneficial skin
- longer fingernails and toenails
- more grounded hair that develops all the more rapidly
- Biotin attempts to energize facial hair development, as well!

Biotin is discovered actually in dairy items, meat, and slick fish, for example, salmon and fish. Likewise nuts, chestnut rice, oats, and avocado. Cheddar, yogurt, chicken, and liver are especially high in biotin. Your hair-grow out of your scalp, which is made of skin. Deal with your skin and you will energize hair development.

Drink eight glasses (64 oz) of water each day.

Eat biotin! You can get it normally by eating nuts, chestnut rice, oats, and different nourishments (see box above.)

Eat nourishments with fundamental unsaturated fats, including walnuts, salmon, and avocado.

Give the collagen that wraps around your hair a help by eating citrus, strawberries, and red peppers. On the other hand take 250 mg of collagen every day.

Verdant green vegetables reinforce your hair follicles by boosting the protein keratin.

Get enough iron by eating red meat, verdant greens, molasses, and dried natural products.

Support your zinc and silica mineral admission with pumpkin seeds, pecans, eggs, shellfish, and cucumber.

Go simple on your hair. Maintain a strategic distance from warmth (level irons, hair curlers, blow driers) and wear your hair up or cover it to shield it from brutal climate.

Biotin Myths and Realities

Biotin is not an enchantment pill. You won't wake up and find that you have transformed into Rapunzel. Your every day biotin supplement is only that, a supplement to your sound eating regimen. Together with great hair mind, these things will offer your hair some assistance with growing longer, quicker.

A few individuals have reported encountering facial break-outs (zits) in the wake of taking biotin, yet there does not appear to be an immediate connection between the biotin and the zits.

Liquor and anti-toxins might keep the body from retaining biotin and obliterate the body's actually delivered B vitamins. On the off chance that you are on a course of anti-infection agents, hold off on your biotin supplements until the anti-toxins are done.

So why do some hair supplements have 5000 mcg and as much as 10,000 mcg of biotin?

Star Tip: You needn't bother with that much – by any stretch of the imagination!

Since it is so natural to acquire our day by day necessity of biotin from our eating regimen (too, our intestinal microorganisms produce biotin – by and large in abundance of our body's day by day needs), there is NO Recommended Dietary Intake (RDI) level. The 'sufficient admission' level – the base sum expected to guarantee that sickness (counting alopecia) connected with lack does not happen – is just 25 micrograms day by day (take note of: this is micrograms, not milligrams). Abundance is essentially dispensed with.

Here are some more actualities about biotin that are going to spare you time, cash, and disillusionment and offer you some assistance with understanding biotin such as a star!

There are eight unique structures (stereoisomers) of biotin, be that as it may, one and only of them is naturally dynamic: d-biotin. This is the structure that is incorporated into our exclusive Biotin recipe.

Biotin helps with numerous metabolic responses, including the creation of solid scalp oils. A lot of or too little oil on the scalp can block or restrain hair development. Biotin enhances the digestion system of scalp oils, making the scalp a more beneficial environment for hair to develop in.

The truth of the matter is, water-dissolvable vitamins, including biotin and other B vitamins, are not put away in the body (dissimilar to fat-solvent vitamins – A, D, E, K – which are put away). Any overabundance – the sum that isn't quickly utilized by the body – is quickly discharged by means of the urinary tract. That is science dialect for 'you pee it out rapidly.' Mega-dosing with biotin is actually flushing your cash down the channel.

You are qualified for thicker, more beneficial, more quickly developing hair, without the big name beautician costs. In case you're worn out on eventual failure marvel prevailing fashions (like biotin) that guarantee you a Beyonce-like coffee, let Hair Essentials and it's clinically demonstrated common equation disentangle your life, and spare you time and cash.

Biotin Can Cure Hair Loss

At the drugstore, you're certain to discover supplements that claim to support your hair and nails. The majority of them contain biotin, which makes up the gathering of B complex vitamins. They have fundamental impact in helping so as to keep up sound hair with digestion system and changing over nourishment for vitality creation. While a biotin inadequacy can trigger balding, an absence of it is really uncommon, as per the Mayo Clinic. "Biotin is just worth taking in case you're having hair breakage issues," Dr. Mercurio says. Despite the fact that it may fortify your hair, there's not solid proof it can do much for male pattern baldness brought about by hormone issues or hereditary qualities. All things considered, you'll likely need a more grounded treatment from your specialist.

In the event that you begin seeing globs of hair in the shower deplete, it's anything but difficult to get ballistic. All things considered, hair can be a critical part of a lady's personality, and male pattern baldness is normally seen as a man's issue. Actually, ladies make up around 40% of the Americans experiencing undesirable shedding, and half of all ladies experience female example male pattern baldness (yes, that exists) by age 50.

So it's a major myth that balding is a man's issue.
Overabundance testosterone does not bring about either sex to go bare—but rather testosterone plays a major part. The body changes over testosterone into dihydrotestosterone (DHT), and this procedure causes harm to the hair follicle, clarifies Dr. Mercurio. So the

individuals who change over testosterone to DHT most effectively lose more hair than those whose bodies are less productive. All things considered, your specialist may endorse a hostile to androgen pharmaceutical to obstruct the impact the hormones have on the hair follicle, says Melissa Piliang, MD, a dermatologist at the Cleveland Clinic in Ohio.

Contraception pills cause male pattern baldness

"Various androgen (male) hormones can cooperate with the hair follicle to make it more slender." Dr. Piliang says. A few sorts of progesterone, a hormone normally found in oral contraceptives, can act like androgens, Dr. Piliang says. Male pattern baldness with the pill is progressively an issue, however, in the event that you're utilizing a more seasoned adaptation of conception prevention. "The fresher ones created have less of those reactions and are truly more hostile to androgen," Dr. Piliang says. Truth be told, a few specialists might recommend conception prevention to battle undesirable male pattern baldness, Dr. Piliang says. Converse with your specialist to locate the right form for you, particularly in the event that you have a family history of balding.

Stress makes your hair drop out

It's anything but difficult to accuse diminishing strands for anxiety, yet for anxiety to bring about male pattern baldness, it must be more compelling than what you encounter when you're preparing for a major presentation at work or in a contention with your life partner. At the point when your body encounters something traumatic, similar to a noteworthy surgery or sickness, it can disturb the cycle of hair, moving it rashly into the shedding stage, Dr. Mercurio says. It's a condition called telogen emanation, which can likewise be created by labor, as per the American Hair Loss Association. Shedding more often than not dies down once the distressing occasion has passed. While a few specialists accept enthusiastic stretch, for example, the passing of a friend or family member can bring about male pattern baldness, nothing has been demonstrated absolutely, Dr. Mercurio says.

All male pattern baldness is changeless

A few cases of shedding could simply be makeshift. Numerous ladies lose some hair subsequent to conceiving an offspring, for occurrence, as their hormones alter back to their pre-pregnancy levels, Dr. Piliang says, however it regrows inside of a while. Numerous ladies likewise have diet issues that influence their hair. "Ladies more regularly than men have nourishing insufficiencies in iron and zinc," Dr. Piliang says. Both are key supplements for solid hair, so low levels could debilitate your strands. You can alter that by expanding your admission of nourishments rich in those supplements, similar to beans and shellfish. You could likewise take supplements, yet check with your specialist first to be sheltered. Best to maintain a strategic distance from compelling eating arranges as well. Any prohibitive eating regimen can prompt hair shedding since you're missing out on vital supplements, Dr. Piliang says.

Food Source of Vitamin H:
Vitamin H can be acquired from nourishments such as vegetables, liver, carrots, brewer's yeast, cooked eggs, cauliflower, oats, mushrooms, nuts, cereal, Bananas, salmon, sardines and soy flour.

1. Digestion system:
Vitamin H is the most indispensable supplement for your metabolic procedure. This procedures all sustenance that you expend like protein, starches, and fat?. Appropriate level of Vitamin H is helpful to handle the nourishment rapidly in the body. Vitamin H supplement can give you alleviation from metabolic issues to work legitimately. This can likewise end up being extremely valuable in weight reduction, as Vitamin H supplement speeds up weight reduction and clear metabolic levels impacts.

2. Glucose:

Vitamin H is imperative for delivering blood glucose in the body. Vitamin H is serves to breakdown starches in the body and keeps up sound glucose levels. Diabetes patients can be encouraged to devour Vitamin H supplement to keep up glucose levels to work appropriately.

3. Hair and Nail Growth:

Vitamin H Hair, Nail Growth Benefits

Vitamin H goes about as the most indispensable component for hair and nails development. Vitamin H insufficiency can bring about male pattern baldness and weak nails. For this situation Vitamin H supplement is encouraged to stop the issue. This vitamin is additionally helpful to support the new development of hair and nail. Standard admission of Vitamin H can be valuable to dispose of this issue.

4. Enhance the soundness of your skin:

Absence of Vitamin H can bring about numerous skin issues like skin inflammation, psoriasis, rashes, dermatitis and irritation. This is likewise essential to help working of the sensory system and hormone capacity. Keeping up appropriate level of Vitamin H levels helps in great skin wellbeing.

5. Help in weight reduction:

Vitamin H is brilliant for legitimate metabolic capacity and helps as a co-compound for nourishment breaking. Vitamin H supports the ideal opportunity for this procedure and separates the nourishment rapidly. This by implication prompts weight reduction, which can be considerably more viable with a sound eating routine and activity administration. This can be the best thinning pill to get your weight reduction objectives.

6. Lower cholesterol:

Vitamin H demonstrates positive result to lower cholesterol that causes coronary illness like heart assault and stroke. Vitamin H is likewise useful in lessening of LDL (terrible cholesterol) levels in the body.

7. Direct glucose:

Vitamin H battles and avoids both sorts of diabetes, type 1 and 2. They give best results when overcome with chromium to fortify glycemic control in hefty with diabetes. Absence of Vitamin H can bring about debilitated glucose resistance and lessening the use of glucose.

8. Pregnancy:

Vitamin H Benefits for Pregnancy

Utilization of Vitamin H can be dealt with as supplement and not sedate. This vitamin can be gotten from the greater part of the nourishment supplement that we expend in our every day diet. Vitamin H has been demonstrated safe for pregnant ladies.

9. Silver hair:

Vitamin H can demonstrate helpful to postpone hair brightening and restore the hormonal parity.

10. Skin wellbeing:

Vitamin H is helpful to keep up hydrated and saturated skin. Stretch imprints and dermatological ailments of the skin such as stretch imprints, vitiligo, skin break out, and dermatitis are brought on by absence of got dried out skin. Vitamin H helps in the skin cell restoration process when consolidated with other B vitamins. They can likewise be joined with numerous different vitamins and minerals like vitamins A, D, E, zinc and unsaturated fats.

11. Cell reinforcements:

Vitamin H is likewise alluded as the "sustaining vitamin", since it is a fundamental cancer prevention agents. Vitamin H acts truly well for cell level, evacuation of poisons and risky gasses that causes cell harm and demise. Vitamin H is valuable to get a solid cell required to flush off the poisons from the body.

12. Wrinkles:

Wrinkles in the middle of eyes and sanctuaries are brought on because of dry wrinkles and expression lines. This is because of loss of fiber cell movement, lessening and crack of collagen strands, neuroendocrine brokenness, and low protein combination rate. It ruins the skin versatility and causes wrinkles. Wrinkles likewise happen because of exorbitant UV radiation, activity and numerous ailments. Biotin is famously utilized by numerous beauty care products businesses to take care of this issues .They are even utilized as a part of BOTOX to explain fishtails lines.

13. Vitamins for Bodybuilders:

Vitamin H Benefits for Body Builders

Biotin helps in the elements of amino corrosive digestion system and produces vitality. This is likewise a decent vitamin for muscle heads that are found in crude egg whites. Eating crude egg whites can bring about development issues and Biotin.

14. Thick mustache:

Thick mustache is an image of manliness and force. This additionally can give an appropriate look to your eyes, button?, and jawbone. Protein-rich foods, minerals and vitamins help in the development rate of hair. A few Deficiencies of vitamins and minerals can postpone your facial hair development. Vitamin H is demonstrated to invigorate sound hair and decrease balding. This can be valuable to get the wanted mustache for guys.

Some imperative tips for Vitamin H:

1. Try not to take dose in substantial amount of Vitamin H supplements.

2. Continuously counsel your specialist before taking Vitamin H supplements.

3. Vitamin H insufficiency can bring about numerous health related issues.

4. Pregnant ladies ought to incorporate said measure of Vitamin H in their eating routine.

5. Common sources are the most ideal approach to acquire Vitamin H.

When buying from us, you should be sure of one thing; we provide the best quality of Vitamin B that can ever be. There will be no traces of any allergic components which most manufacturers add as a source of preservation. We preserve our vitamins the natural way.

Consult with your physician if you experience excessive hair fall even after a month or two of starting Biotin. If Biotin deficiency is your reason of hair fall, it will definitely be decreased in two week's time.

Cheers to long and luscious locks when buying from us.

www.ingramcontent.com/pod-product-compliance
Lightning Source LLC
Chambersburg PA
CBHW081541280526
45788CB00010B/3321